Sandra Regina De Magalhães
Andréia Vieira Pereira
Carmem Patrícia Barbosa

Cardiovascular diseases

AF303838

Sandra Regina De Magalhães
Andréia Vieira Pereira
Carmem Patrícia Barbosa

Cardiovascular diseases

Evaluation of visitors to a scientific exhibition on Human Anatomy

ScienciaScripts

Imprint

Any brand names and product names mentioned in this book are subject to trademark, brand or patent protection and are trademarks or registered trademarks of their respective holders. The use of brand names, product names, common names, trade names, product descriptions etc. even without a particular marking in this work is in no way to be construed to mean that such names may be regarded as unrestricted in respect of trademark and brand protection legislation and could thus be used by anyone.

Cover image: www.ingimage.com

This book is a translation from the original published under ISBN 978-620-2-04046-4.

Publisher:
Sciencia Scripts
is a trademark of
Dodo Books Indian Ocean Ltd. and OmniScriptum S.R.L publishing group

120 High Road, East Finchley, London, N2 9ED, United Kingdom
Str. Armeneasca 28/1, office 1, Chisinau MD-2012, Republic of Moldova, Europe
Printed at: see last page
ISBN: 978-620-7-21295-8

Copyright © Sandra Regina De Magalhães, Andréia Vieira Pereira, Carmem Patrícia Barbosa
Copyright © 2024 Dodo Books Indian Ocean Ltd. and OmniScriptum S.R.L publishing group

CONTENTS

ACKNOWLEDGMENTS

First of all, we thank God who allowed us to overcome difficulties and carry out this project, not as a solo effort, but with the participation of special people in our lives.

We would also like to thank the State University of Maringà (UEM) and the UEM Dynamic Interdisciplinary Museum (MUDI) for the friendly and creative environment they offer to all their students. We would also like to express our gratitude to the Pro-Rector of Extension and Culture (PEC) and to Professor Dr. Itana Maria de Souza Gimenes for their support. We would like to thank Professor Dr. Marcilio Hubner de Miranda Neto, as the founder and maintainer of MUDI-UEM, and Professor Dr. Ana Paula Vidotti, as the coordinator of MUDI-UEM, for the opportunity to hold the exhibition and the research within this non-formal educational space that has benefited so many people, not only from the academic community, but also from the outside community.

To the Department of Morphological Sciences (DCM) at UEM and all its teaching staff for their dedication and for building not only cognitive learning, but also as a manifestation of the affective nature of education in the process of *professional training*. Special *mention goes* to Professor Dr. Josiane Medeiros de Mello and the DCM technical team who influenced, collaborated and dedicated part of their knowledge and activities to making the exhibition a reality. Our sincere gratitude goes to Marcelo Vlademir Piloto, Liana Ribeiro Zanzarini, Maria Vilma Moraes de Sarro, Reinaldo de Castro Soriani and Joâo Batista.

To my colleagues from the Anatomy and Histology postgraduate course at DCM-UEM, André Felipe Paixâo - for contributing to and producing the educational video shown to visitors during the exhibition, Diogo Rodrigues Jimenes, Ryan Palhano Gonzales Pompalino, Gracielle Baraviera Scardelato and André Luis Schimidt da Silva - for their constant support in setting up the entire exhibition.

We would also like to thank Mrs. Aparecida do Carmo Gaviolli and Mrs. Elizângela Cristina Magalhaes who, in addition to their emotional support, helped to improve the aesthetic aspects of the exhibition and helped us a lot in times of difficulty.

Finally, we would like to thank all the researchers and authors whose work has been referenced in this book, as many have contributed to the success of this work.

AUTHORS' BIOGRAPHIES

Sandra Regina de Magalhaes

She has a degree in Aesthetics and Cosmetics Technology from the Centro Universitàrio de Maringà (Unicesumar), a specialist degree in Anatomy and Histology from the Universidade Estadual de Maringà (UEM) and a post-graduate degree in Higher Education Teaching from the Centro Universitàrio de Maringà (Unicesumar). She currently works with personalized client care in the areas of facial, body and therapeutic aesthetics.

Andreia Vieira Pereira

Veterinary Doctor graduated from the Federal University of Campina Grande (2007); Master in Zootechnics with emphasis on Pharmacology and Toxicology of Natural Products, from the Federal University of Campina Grande (2010); PhD in Tropical Diseases from the Botucatu Medical School/UNESP (2013); Post-doctoral student in Experimental Pathology at the State University of Londrina (2014-2017).

Carmen Patricia Barbosa

He has a degree in Physiotherapy from the State University of Londrina (1997), a specialization in Morphophysiology Applied to Body Education and Rehabilitation from the State University of Maringà (2000), a master's degree (2002) and a doctorate (2015) in Biological Sciences from the State University of Maringà, in the area of Cell Biology.

She was a professor of Human Anatomy, Human Physiology, Neurofunctional Bases of Movement and Kinesiology and Biomechanics at the Maringà Higher Education Center (UniCesumar) from 2002 to 2015, and since 2012 she has been a professor of Human Anatomy at the Department of Morphological Sciences (DCM) of the State University of Maringà.

She has teaching experience in all health courses, both at undergraduate and postgraduate level. She is a researcher, advisor and author of books in her field, and is on the editorial board of important scientific journals.

The field of education is quite vast, since education takes place in many places: in the family, at work, on the street, in the factory, in the media, in politics and *also* at school (PIMENTA, 1999).

1. INTRODUCTION

This study aimed to assess the level of knowledge of visitors to a scientific exhibition about the circulatory system and the main aspects of cardiovascular diseases such as etiology, signs, symptoms, forms of treatment, diagnostic methods and preventive aspects. The exhibition was held from December 2016 to February 2017 at the Dynamic Interdisciplinary Museum (MUDI) of the State University of Maringà (UEM), in partnership with the Department of Morphological Sciences (DCM) of UEM, in the area of Human Anatomy. The entire experimental protocol was previously approved by UEM's Permanent Committee for Ethics in Research with Human Beings (COPEP) (under CAAE n° 63021616.0.0000.0104 and final approval protocol n° 1.897.921).

Visitors over the age of 18, of both sexes, were approached at random and voluntarily agreed to sign an informed consent form and take part in the research by filling in a questionnaire while visiting the exhibition. This survey instrument was drawn up by the researchers responsible for this study and previously validated by three other professors from the DCM who are renowned researchers.

Although research is being carried out to reduce the incidence, morbidity and mortality of cardiovascular diseases and although there are now modern diagnostic techniques and treatments for these diseases, they still represent a major challenge for public health worldwide. This is because, among many other implications, they negatively affect the country's productivity and tend to increase as a result of rising life expectancy and an ageing population. For this reason, they must be viewed by the competent authorities with a great deal of discretion and rigor, and must be seen as one of the great future challenges for developing countries.

In Brazil, for example, a number of action plans and strategies to tackle cardiovascular diseases and their associated ailments have been put into practice in recent years by the Ministry of Health, with the aim of promoting changes in daily habits that improve the population's quality of life (BRASIL, 2012). In addition, low-cost educational actions and early intervention can promote the dissemination of preventive measures for many of the ailments associated with them.

In this context, teaching and research institutions play a crucial role in the Ministry of Health, since they must act as producers, promoters and disseminators of knowledge. Thus, the effective action of these institutions must be able to promote the dissemination of basic knowledge to the general population, which does not always have access to relevant information in an accessible language.

For all the above reasons, the relevance of this study lies in the fact that we believe in the importance of disseminating knowledge as the main preventive measure capable of minimizing the damage caused by cardiovascular diseases. Furthermore, we believe that investing in dissemination can reduce complications and even minimize the costly public expenditure on curative and palliative treatments. Thus, we hope that this study can contribute relevant information for the application of new public policies to be adopted preventively in order to minimize the incidence and serious consequences of cardiovascular diseases in Brazil.

Keywords: Circulatory system; heart; hypertension; cardiovascular disease prevention; public health.

2. BRIEF THEORETICAL REVIEW

The search for knowledge about the anatomy and physiology of the circulatory system (CS) is not new; on the contrary, it has progressed with great interest since ancient times. There are reports, for example, that in ancient Egypt, around 3500 BC, people believed that elements such as urine, air, blood and even the soul itself circulated within vessels that were connected to the heart. However, a few years later, with scientific advances and the possibility of performing anatomical dissections of the human body, it was discovered that only blood circulated in these vessels, which were then called arteries and veins. Galen thus effectively proved that the arteries contained only blood and not air or any other compound. In addition, more specific morphological studies showed that arteries were around six times thicker than veins (BESTETTI, RESTINI and COUTO, 2014).

Later, another great scholar on the subject and considered by many to be the "father of modern anatomy", Andreas Vesalius, made great discoveries that improved other researchers' understanding of the subject. One of them, the physician William Harvey, was specifically interested in the anatomy of the heart and blood vessels, as well as the forces capable of generating the movements that made the blood flow inside the vessels. His work was essential for understanding the mechanisms that trigger blood circulation (HART, 2001).

Nowadays, many anatomical dissection studies, functional, clinical, laboratory and experimental studies have led to a broad understanding of all the structures that make up and all the factors that influence this intriguing system. Silverthorn (2010), for example, points out that the CS is formed by the heart which, as a central organ, acts like a propulsive contractile pump capable of propelling blood through a series of tubular structures of different diameters known as blood vessels. Thus, through this closed system of tubes, blood circulates throughout the body, reaching all its parts in order to distribute nutrients and oxygen necessary for cellular irrigation. Likewise, this same mechanism allows the drainage of waste materials produced by the cells, so that the homeostasis of the environment is maintained.

Alongside the evolution of studies applied to the anatomy and physiology of the CS, there has also been a growing and progressive interest in better understanding the study of diseases that affect this system. In this way, pathology applied to the CS has made it possible to elucidate the etiology, related risk factors, epidemiological factors, pathophysiological mechanisms, as well as preventive and curative treatments for the main diseases involving it (BRASILEIRO FILHO et al., 2016).

Thus, among the various chronic non-communicable diseases (NCDs) currently being studied and which have represented a major challenge to public health worldwide, cardiovascular diseases (CVDs) are included, which are accompanied by high rates of hospital admissions, physical disabilities and even deaths. According to Villela, Klein and Oliveira (2016), in 2010 alone there were 35 million deaths worldwide associated with these diseases. According to these authors, this number continues to grow exponentially and additionally, data from the Unified Health System (SUS) reveals that more than 28% of deaths in Brazil in 2012 alone were attributed to CVDs.

Among the various diseases that can be classified as cardiovascular, the most common include hypertension, atherosclerosis, heart failure and acute myocardial infarction. However, peripheral vascular disease, cerebrovascular accidents (formerly known as strokes), aneurysms, endocarditis and myocarditis also complete this picture (BONOW et al., 2013).

Of all these diseases, hypertension stands out, as it occurs so frequently that it affects one in five people in the world, with 15% to 20% of the Brazilian population considered to be hypertensive. In addition, if not treated properly, it can lead to the rupture of important blood vessels and be associated with strokes or heart failure. Therefore, if hypertension is not controlled, it triggers metabolic alterations, hormonal changes and vascular hypertrophy (FERREIRA and AYDOS, 2010).

Another CVD to be highlighted is atherosclerosis, whose studies published by the World Health Organization (WHO) define it as a set of alterations deriving from the accumulation of lipids, calcium and fibrous connective tissue in the intima layer of the arteries. Thus, in this disease, the arteries suffer severe structural degradation, causing a loss of their natural elasticity and a reduction in their caliber. These changes progressively reduce systemic blood flow, compromising tissues and organs that need constant and uninterrupted blood supply, such as the heart and brain. For this reason, when atherosclerosis affects one of the coronary arteries, for example, the individual can develop heart failure or even acute myocardial infarction (NETO, 2008).

According to Mussi and Pereira (2010), in myocardial infarction there is necrosis of the heart muscle due to a lack of adequate nutrition and, in 25% of cases, death is inevitable. This is because the time elapsed between the onset of cardiac hypoxia and tissue damage is very short, making rescue impossible in most cases. Although the high mortality rates related to myocardial infarction can be reduced by prompt treatment, unfortunately the vast majority of people do not recognize its initial signs and symptoms, making immediate help impossible.

A major aggravating factor related to these diseases is the fact that, in the majority of cases, they affect and cause death in people over 30 years of age, negatively affecting the country's productivity and should therefore be viewed very strictly by the authorities. Furthermore, reversing this situation seems difficult, as an increase in the prevalence of CVDs has been described concomitantly with an increase in life expectancy and an ageing population. For this reason, one of the great challenges for developing countries is to reconcile the process of population ageing with scientific and technological developments in the health area capable of facilitating early diagnosis and favoring specific treatments for such diseases (MANSUR and FAVORATO, 2016). It is important to emphasize that, although primary aging is inevitable and determined by genetics, secondary aging (which results from external influences and is variable among individuals) and tertiary or terminal aging (which is marked by profound physical and cognitive losses) can be avoided or even mitigated (FECCHINE and TROMPIERI, 2012).

According to Brisciliari et al. (2014), the correlation between the increase in the incidence of CVDs and population ageing is related to the significant improvement in the quality of life of the population in general and their easier access to health services. Thus, as the population ages, the prevalence of CVD increases, with estimates pointing to the fact that by the year 2020 there will be an increase of around 15% in the number of deaths from CVD worldwide. For this reason, authors such as Trapè et.al. (2014) emphasize that the authorities' main concern should not be with the growing number of elderly people, but rather with the way in which this population will age, since ageing is strongly associated with structural and functional changes in bodily structures. Ferreti, Mattiello and Teo Arruda (2014), for example, point out that these changes have been exhaustively studied in order to better understand susceptibility to the development of chronic illnesses that compromise quality of life and make people vulnerable to acquiring diseases.

This issue is becoming even more relevant in developing countries, as estimates point to the fact that by 2050, the population over the age of 65 will double, representing a major challenge for these countries. This is because public spending to specifically meet the demands of this population (with social benefits, pensions and adequate health treatment conditions) is significant and even greater when this stage of life is not accompanied by physical and mental health (LEITE et al., 2015). For this reason, according to Malta and Silva-Jùnior (2013), common illnesses at this age entail significant costs not only for the patient themselves, but also for family members and the state.

In Brazil, it has been found that two-thirds of deaths are related to CNCDs, especially CVDs (MAIA and CUNHA, 2014) and that, to make matters worse, these diseases mostly affect people with lower purchasing power, low levels of education, little access to information and quality health services (MALTA and SILVA-JÙNIOR, 2013). In addition, according to Viera et al. (2016), the information department of the Unified Health System (DATASUS) reports that expenses related to NCDs in Brazil are very high, generating a significant impact on the budgets of health funding bodies. This is the case, for example, with the cost of hospital services in the northeastern region of the country between January 2008 and July 2015, which was equivalent to R$ 2,460,057,417.04 and in the state of Bahia, which represented an expense of R$ 579,984,470.55.

According to Muniz and collaborators (2012), smoking, poor diet and a sedentary lifestyle are some of the main causes of CNCDs, and obesity and overweight in the population can be considered a global epidemic. This concern was confirmed by data released by the Vigitel survey (Surveillance of Risk and Protective Factors for Chronic Diseases by Telephone Survey), which pointed out that while in 2006 the number of overweight Brazilians was 42.5%, in 2012 this figure rose to 52.8%. Also according to recent studies by the State University of Rio de Janeiro (UERJ) based on relative risks (international data) and the obesity index in Brazil, it is estimated that the SUS spends R$2.37 billion a year on cardiovascular diseases resulting from complications of obesity in the population, and that the estimated costs correspond to around 0.1% of the national GDP in 2010 (BAHIA E ARAÙJO, 2014).

The high rates of overweight have attracted the attention of researchers and health professionals in Brazil and around the world. It is estimated that between 40% and 80% of individuals who were overweight during adolescence are prone to obesity in adulthood. Unfortunately, in 2012, when 45,900 adults were assessed in Brazil, it was found that 51% of them were overweight and 17% were obese (MARTINS, 2013). Although the figures are indeed frightening, many factors related to obesity and CVD are perfectly modifiable and should be known by the general population so that harmful daily habits can be modified and these diseases prevented.

As such, there is a great need to develop educational actions and effective, low-cost, preventive interventions that favor the early diagnosis and treatment of NCDs. According to Brasil (2012), some action plans with strategies for tackling them have already been put into practice in Brazil in recent years by the Ministry of Health, with the aim of promoting changes in daily habits that improve the population's quality of life. According to Malta and Silva-Jùnior (2013), this plan of strategic actions for tackling CNCDs by 2022 will address the four main groups of these diseases: diseases of the circulatory system, cancer, chronic respiratory diseases and diabetes. In addition, it will address the main risk factors for CNCDs, such as smoking, harmful alcohol consumption, physical inactivity, poor diet and obesity.

In this regard, the Ministry of Health is counting on the help and participation of the country's teaching and research institutions, as producers and promoters of knowledge. This is because it is believed that investing in publicizing the prevention of the main risk factors that lead to so many complications is of fundamental importance (FERRETI, MATTIELLO E ARRUDA, 2014). Therefore, the aim of this study was to inform visitors to a scientific exhibition held at a higher education institution about the basic aspects of CH and various factors related to CVD. It also aimed to assess the level of knowledge of visitors to the exhibition about the main CVDs in terms of their signs and symptoms, etiology, diagnostic methods, forms of treatment and preventive aspects. It is hoped that the profile portrayed here can contribute relevant information for the application of new public policies to be adopted in a mainly preventive manner in order to minimize the incidence and serious consequences of these diseases in Brazil.

3. MATERIALS AND METHODS

This study was carried out during a scientific exhibition entitled "Anatomical Exhibition of Human Hearts at the Dynamic Interdisciplinary Museum (MUDI) of the State University of Maringà (UEM)", which took place between December 2016 and February 2017.

The entire experimental protocol described below was previously approved by the UEM Permanent Committee for Ethics in Research with Human Beings (COPEP), under protocol no. 63021616.0.0000.0104, with final approval protocol no. 1.897.921.

During this event, visitors to the exhibition were shown healthy and diseased anatomical specimens specially dissected for this purpose.

In this way, normal and pathological human hearts were exhibited, as well as pieces showing the *in situ* location of the heart and the large blood vessels of the body. Synthetic specimens were used, including a human fetus dissected and preserved in glycerin, and a block containing the lungs, mediastinal organs, heart and great vessels of an adult. In addition, special techniques for preparing anatomical specimens (known as angiotechniques) were presented, as well as three optical microscopes with previously focused slides showing the differentiation of arteries and veins and microscopic details of the cardiac striated muscle (myocardium).

Secondly, visitors were introduced to a range of relevant information about the main CVDs in terms of their signs and symptoms, etiology, diagnostic methods, forms of treatment and preventive aspects. Visitors were also able to watch a video explaining these topics, which had been specially prepared for the event in question. The attendance of all the visitors was recorded in a Minute Book, which is held by MUDI-UEM.

Finally, visitors of both sexes who were over 18 years of age at the time of the visit were randomly invited to fill in a survey instrument to analyze their knowledge of factors related to the main CVDs. An investigative questionnaire drawn up by the researchers responsible for the study and previously validated by three other UEM professors (Annex 1) was used to assess the main aspects of these diseases, such as etiology, signs and symptoms, diagnostic and therapeutic methods, and preventive factors. The questionnaire was answered immediately after the visit and handed in to the researchers.

However, before the subjects filled in the questionnaire, they were informed about the aims of the study and how it would be carried out. Thus, the age of majority and voluntary participation were the only criteria for inclusion and exclusion in this study, so that those interested voluntarily signed the Free and Informed Consent Form (Appendix 2) and then completed the questionnaire.

After collecting the data, the questionnaires were tabulated and interpreted considering the mean ± standard error, and graphs and tables were prepared using the *GraphPad Prism software* (version 5). A 95% confidence interval was used.

4. RESULTS

4.1 General aspects of the scientific exhibition

External and internal curtains were specially made for the exhibition, and the color red was chosen to induce visitors to associate it with the color of blood. *Banners*, shelves to hold the anatomical specimens and supports for the microscopes and the Minute Book were also prepared for this event (Figures 1 and 2).

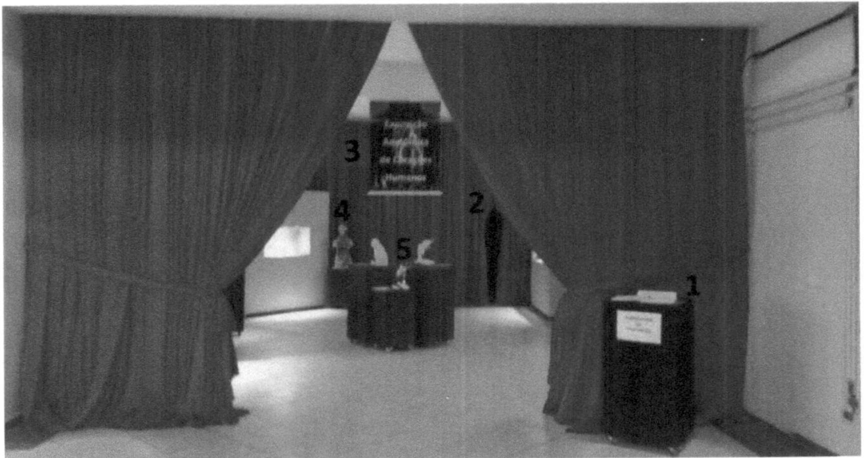

Figura 1. External overview of the scientific exhibition on human hearts at MUDI-UEM.

1 : Minute book for visitors to sign the attendance list; 2: Cinema where the instructional video was shown; 3: *Banner* with the name of the scientific exhibition; 4: Synthetic stem used to identify the location of the heart and great vessels *in the* human body *in situ*; 5: Optical microscopes used to show histological slides of the cardiac striated muscle and the differentiation of arteries and veins.

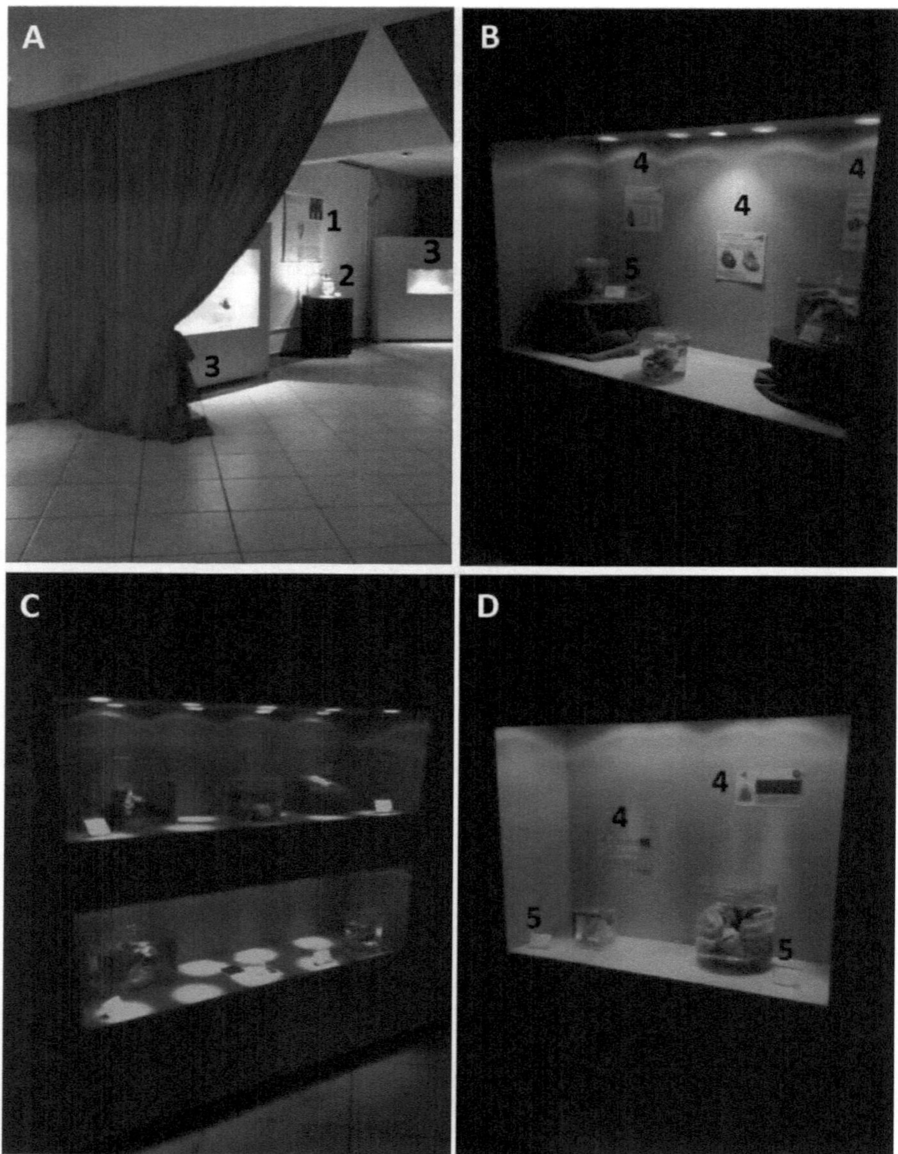

Figura 2. A: View of the left side of the scientific exhibition on human hearts at MUDI-UEM. 1: Information *banner* on the exhibition theme; 2: Human heart with special lighting; 3: Shelves where the dissected pieces were displayed. **B, C** and **D**: Front view of the shelves where the dissected pieces were displayed. Note the different lighting in each room. 4: *Banners* with theoretical information about each specimen on display; 5: Labels identifying the specimen, the technique

used to prepare it and the name of the professional technician responsible for its preparation.

4.2 Anatomical parts for identifying the *in situ* location of the heart and great vessels of the human body

A synthetic torso, a human fetus and a block of organs were used to show the *in situ* location of the heart and the main blood vessels in the human body (Figure 3). All the details numbered in Figure 3 were explained by means of theoretical explanations by the exhibition monitors and illustrative *banners* on the subject.

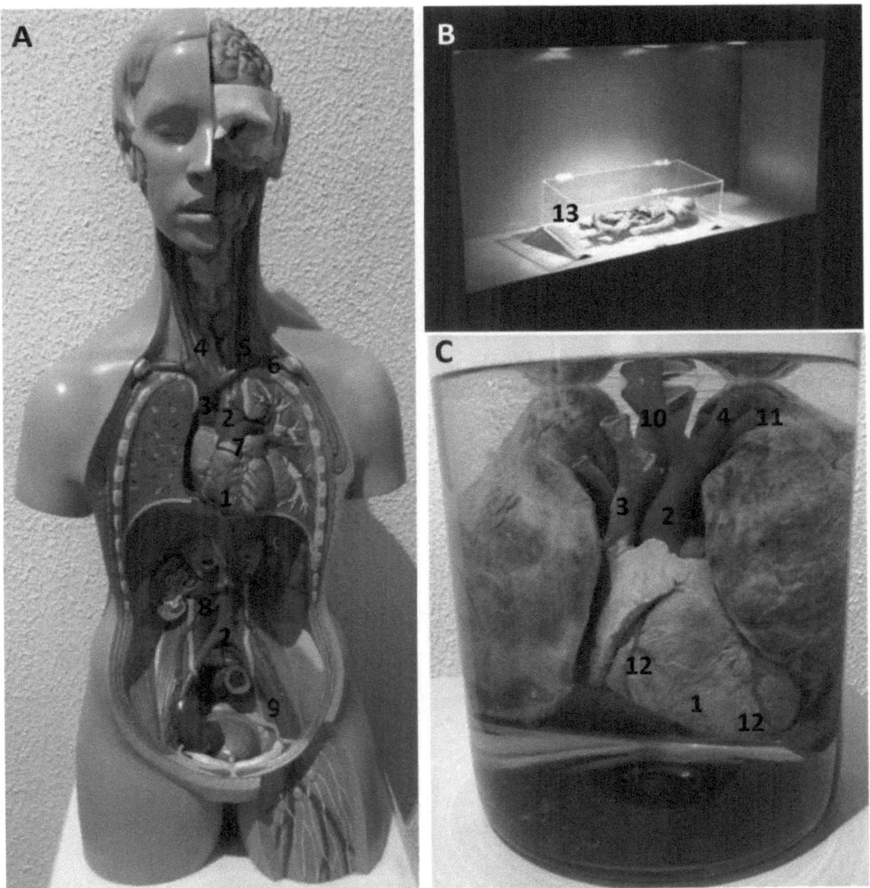

Figure 3. A: Synthetic trunk. **B:** Human fetus preserved in glycerin (upper lateral view). **C:** Block of organs from an adult preserved in formaldehyde. All these pieces were used to show the *in situ*

location of the heart and the large blood vessels of the body. 1: Location of the heart in the mediastinal region; 2: A. aorta; 3: V. superior cava; 4: A. common carotid; 5: V. external jugular; 6: V. subclavian; 7: Pulmonary trunk; 8: V. inferior vena cava; 9: Common iliac artery and vena; 10: Brachiocephalic trunk; 11: Subclavian artery; 12: Branches of the coronary arteries; 13: Acrylic box for storing the fetus. A. Artery; V. Vein.

4.3 Healthy anatomical parts

The hearts of adults and children were exposed to show anatomical structures such as auricles, ventricles, fibrous pericardium, myocardium and great vessels (Figure 4).

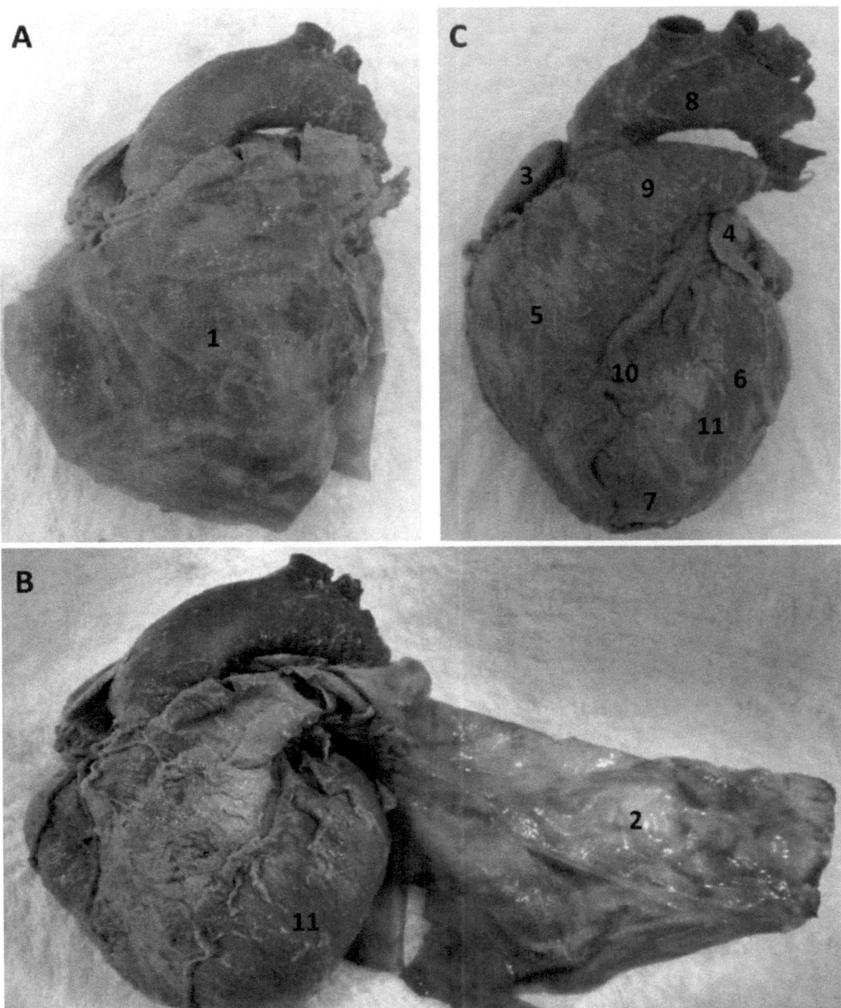

Figure 4. A: Heart covered by fibrous pericardium (1). **B**: Heart with the fibrous pericardium dissected and laterally folded (2). **C:** Heart without the fibrous pericardium showing the right atrium (3), left atrium (4), right ventricle (5), left ventricle (6), apex of the heart (7), aortic artery (8), pulmonary trunk (9) and coronary artery (10). In **B** and **C,** the muscular makeup of the heart is clearly visible (cardiac striated muscle / myocardium; 11).

Two normal adult hearts were exposed to show the heart valves. One of them was cut in coronal section (Figure 5A) and the other at the level of the atria (Figure 5B) to expose and theoretically explain the structures acting in the heart valve mechanism.

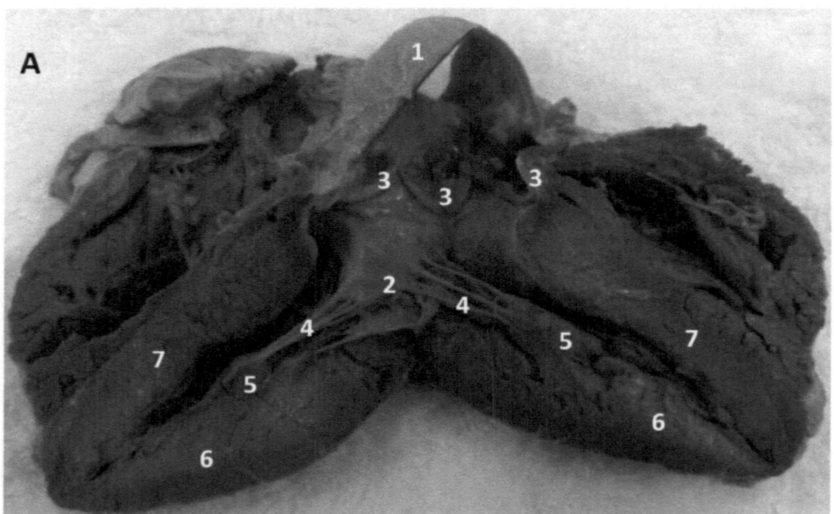

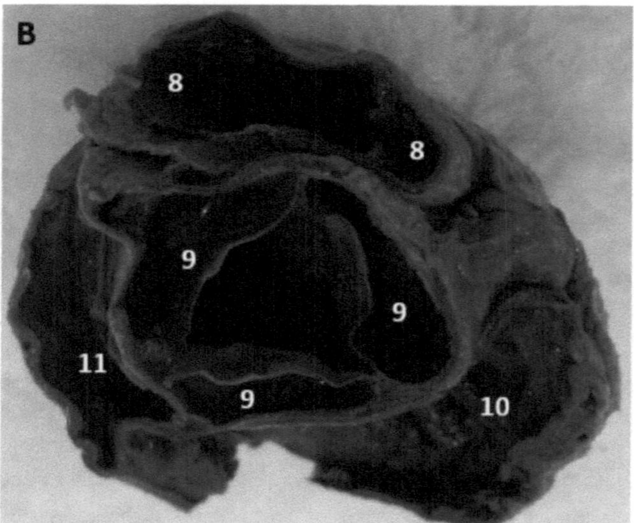

Figure 5. A: Coronal section of the heart showing: sectioned aortic artery (1), connective tissue constituting one of the heart valves (2), seminular valves of the aortic artery (3), chordae tendineae (4), papillary muscles (5). The entire muscular structure of the heart (myocardium; 6) and the interventricular septum (7) were evidenced. B Heart Sectioned at the level of the atria, seen from above. Note the semilunar valves of the pulmonary trunk (8), the semilunar valves of the aortic

artery (9), the right (10) and left (11) atrioventricular ostia.

4.4 Diseased anatomical parts

After a theoretical and practical explanation of the location, anatomy, physiology and general aspects of the heart and great vessels, the visitors were taken to a section of the exhibition where only pathological anatomical specimens were shown. In this context, they were able to see human hearts with saphenous vein grafts, Chagas' disease, cardiac tamponade, heart surgery, myocardial ischemia and heart valve replacement surgery.

Figure 6 shows an adult heart preserved in formaldehyde and sectioned from the coronal plane to show severe myocardial ischemia. When this piece was presented to the visitors, the concept of acute myocardial infarction was discussed, as well as its pathophysiology, which basically results from the obstruction of the coronary arteries and their main branches, leading to an imbalance between oxygen supply and consumption, predisposing to necrosis or cell death (BRANDI, 2017).

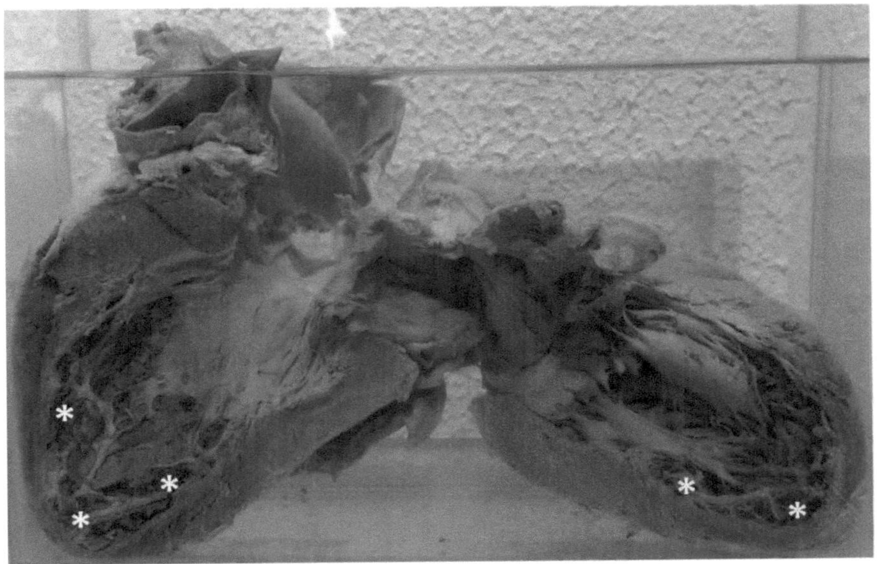

Figure 6. Coronal section of the heart showing an extensive area of myocardial ischemia (*).

In addition, two hearts that had undergone surgical procedures were presented. In one of them (Figure 7A), it was possible to identify the suture on the external portion of the myocardium. In another (Figure 7B), it was possible to see a valvular prosthesis.

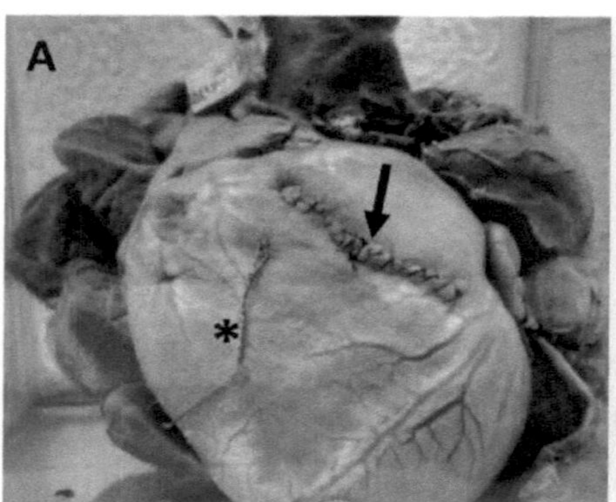
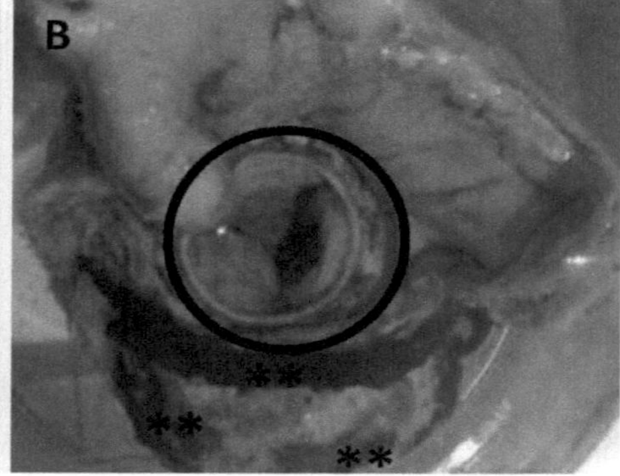

Figure 7. Pathological human hearts submitted to heart surgery. **A**: Frontal view of the heart showing the suture on the external portion of the myocardium (arrow). **B**: Top view of the heart showing the implanted valve prosthesis (inside the circle). *Cardiac vessels stained blue (to show veins) and red (to show arteries).

When these parts were presented to the visitors, the valvular mechanism of the heart was discussed, as well as the possible surgical corrections that can be performed in the case of congenital or acquired diseases that specifically affect the heart valve system. Thus, the mechanical and biological heart valve prostheses were theoretically exposed, as well as the criteria for choice that should be considered individually, such as the biological prosthesis, which is contraindicated for patients in the growth phase (MACIEL E NETO, 2005).

In addition, a heart undergoing bypass surgery (Figure 8A), a heart with Chagas' disease (Figure 8B) and a heart with cardiac tamponade (Figure 8C) were presented and explained to the visitors.

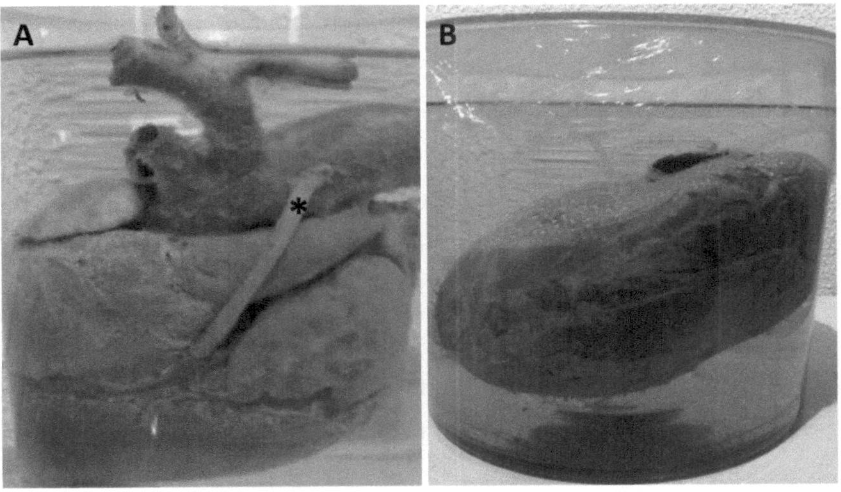

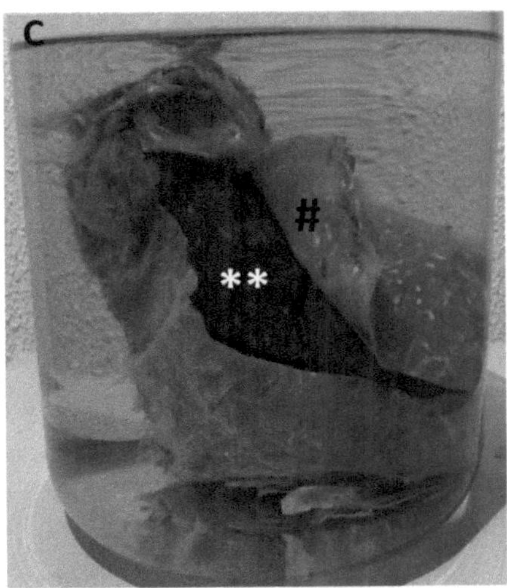

Figure 8: Pathological human hearts. **A**: Heart with surgical repair (saphenous vein bypass*). **B**: Heart showing

cardiomegaly due to Chagas' disease. **C**: Heart with fibrous pericardium (#) dissected and laterally rebated to show cardiac tamponade (**). It is worth noting that it is impossible to see the myocardium due to the accumulation of blood between the myocardium and the pericardium.

When the piece with the saphenous vein bypass was presented, it was emphasized that this procedure consists of a graft performed on the obstructed coronary artery using the person's own great saphenous vein with the aim of re-establishing the perfusion of the obstructed vessel and thus preserving the integrity of the myocardium. It was also emphasized that coronary artery bypass grafting has been considered the most tested surgical procedure in the history of medicine and that it was first proposed in 1967 by the Argentine surgeon René Favaloro and has since represented a major revolution in cardiological therapy (QUINTANA and KALLIL, 2012).

In the Chagas' disease piece, it was emphasized that this disease is considered a tissue and blood parasitosis, whose etiological agent *Trypanosoma (Schizotrypanum) cruzi* transmits it to humans through their feces. Thus, the parasite induces three main pathological processes: exacerbated inflammatory response, cell damage and tissue fibrosis in various organs, most frequently in the heart, digestive system and nervous system (BESTETTI, BARALDI and RESTINI, 2016).

Finally, in the piece with cardiac tamponade, it was stated that this disease results from the accumulation of liquid (mainly blood) between the two membranes of the pericardium, so that the heart loses its contractile capacity and its action of pumping blood to the organs of the body (DAVIDSON, 2001).

4.5 Differentiated anatomical techniques

Different techniques were used to prepare special anatomical pieces that would allow direct observation and study of the structures of the circulatory system in a three-dimensional way, which is essential for learning. Thus, arterial vessels were marked in silver by injecting mercury (Figures 9A and 10C), in blue or beige latex (Figures 9B and 10A), and the heart chambers and vessels at the base of the heart were exposed using the repletion technique (Figures 9B and 10B).

According to Eloi et al. (2010) and Rodrigues et al. (1999), angiotechniques are used to fill blood vessels with coloured, radiopaque or mercurial solutions, helping to study the vascularization of organs and tissues, and have been especially used in the study of cardiac vascularization and the morphology of coronary arteries. Diaphanization and corrosion aim to create models in which blood vessels and heart chambers can be perfectly visualized.

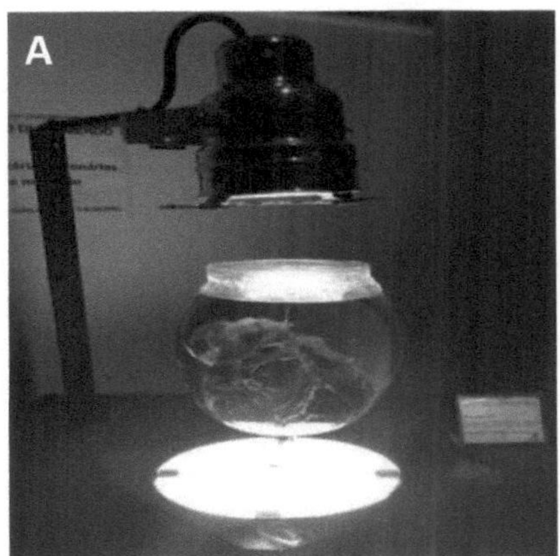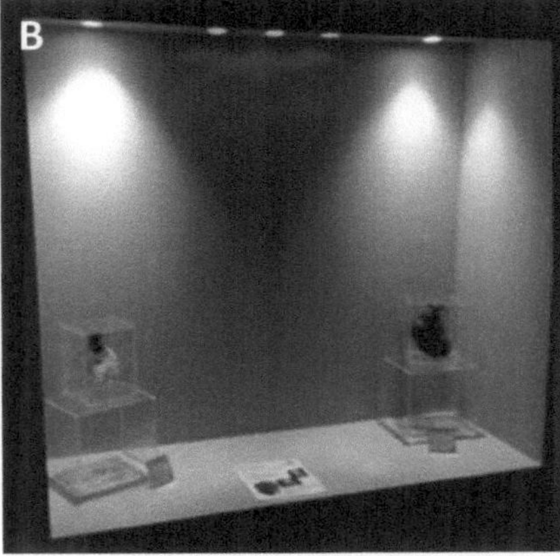

Figure 9. A: Human heart prepared by diaphanization. Note the special lighting, the transparency of the atria and the branches of the coronary arteries injected with mercury. **B**: General view of two specimens prepared using the filling technique followed by the injection of colored latex to identify the coronary arteries and their main branches, as well as the heart chambers.

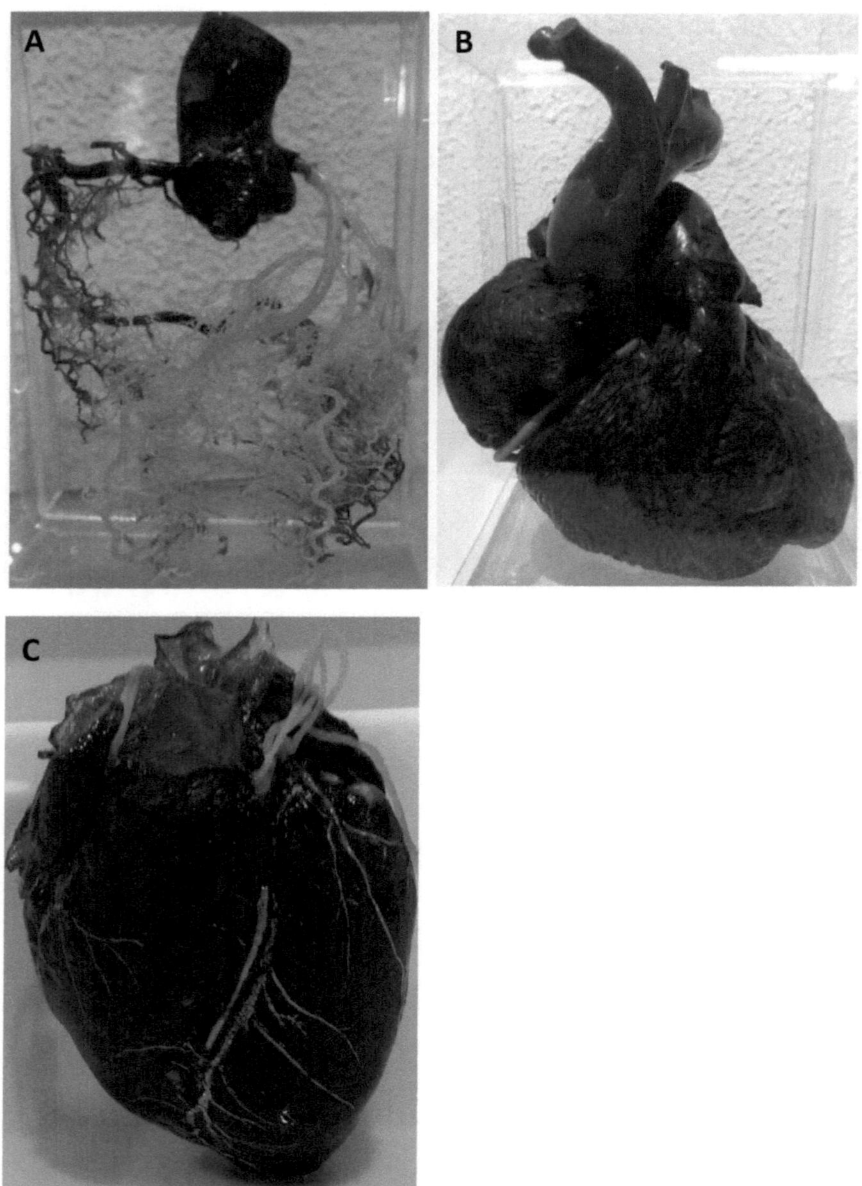

Figure 10A and **10B:** Highlight of the pieces shown in figure 9B. **C**: Highlight of the piece shown in figure 9A.

1.6 Photomicrographs of histological slides of blood vessels and heart

Figures 11, 12, 13 and 14 are photomicrographs taken using a microscope with high-resolution image capture (Olympus Digital Trinocular CX31®). For Figures 11, 12 and 13, the magnifications were 2x (in the images on the left) and 4x (in the images on the right). For Figure 14, both magnifications were 20x.

All the histological slides of blood vessels and cardiac striated muscle (myocardium) shown in Figures 11, 12, 13 and 14 were stained using the Hematoxylin-Eosin (H.E.), Verhoeff or Van Geison staining techniques, and were viewed by visitors to the scientific exhibition using optical microscopes.

While Figure 11 shows the peculiarities of an elastic artery, Figure 12 shows the microscopic structure of a muscular artery and Figure 13 that of a vein. Finally, Figure 14 shows a detailed view of the myocardium of the left ventricle (in cross-section) as well as a congested blood vessel supplying it.

Before the visits, the technicians in charge of the exhibition would place the slides and highlight the structures to be shown, such as the intima, media and adventitia of the vessels, and the cells and vessels of the myocardium.

Figure 11

HISTOLOGICAL SECTIONS

ELASTIC ARTERY

HEMATOXYLIN-EOSIN STAINING TECHNIQUE

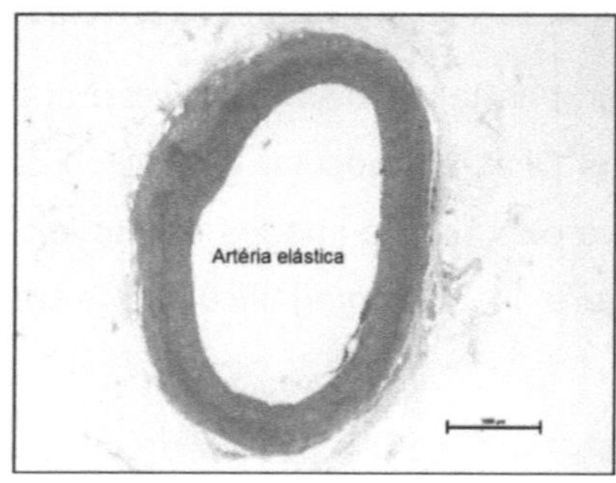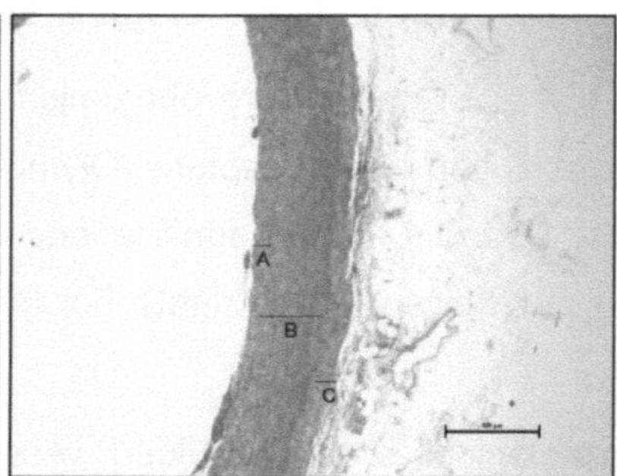

Elastic art

(A)Intimate tunic.

(B)Medium, thick tunic, composed of organized elastic fibres.

(C)Adventitious technique.

VERHOEFF STAINING TECHNIQUE

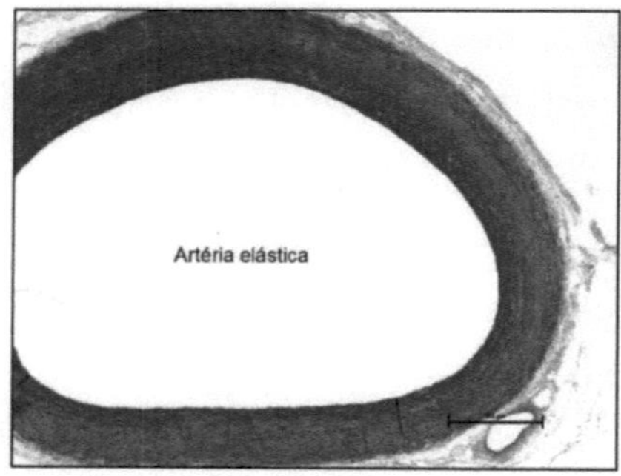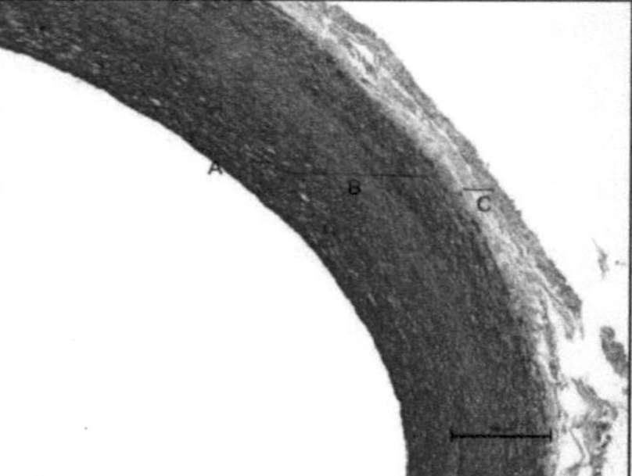

Elastic art

(A)Intimate tunic.

(B)Medium, thick tunic, composed of organized elastic fibres.

(C)Adventitious technique.

Figure 12

HISTOLOGICAL SECTIONS

MUSCULAR ARTERY

HEMATOXYLIN-EOSIN STAINING TECHNIQUE

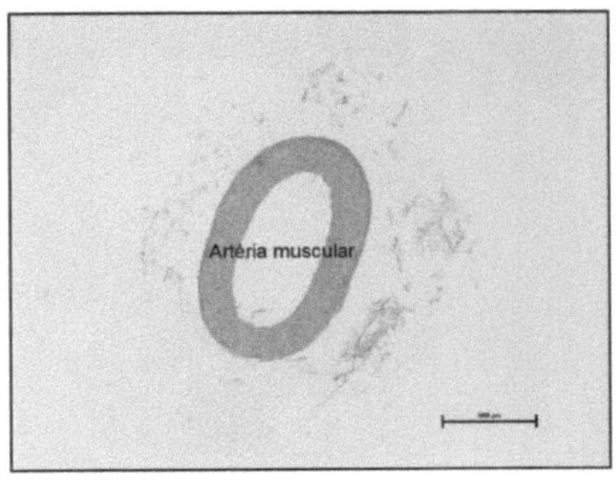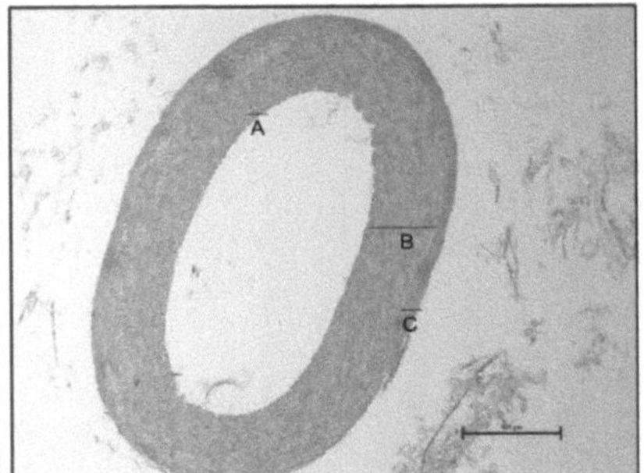

Elastic art

(A)Intimate tunic.

(B)Medium, thick tunic, composed of organized elastic fibres.

(C)Adventitious technique.

VAN GEISON STAINING TECHNIQUE

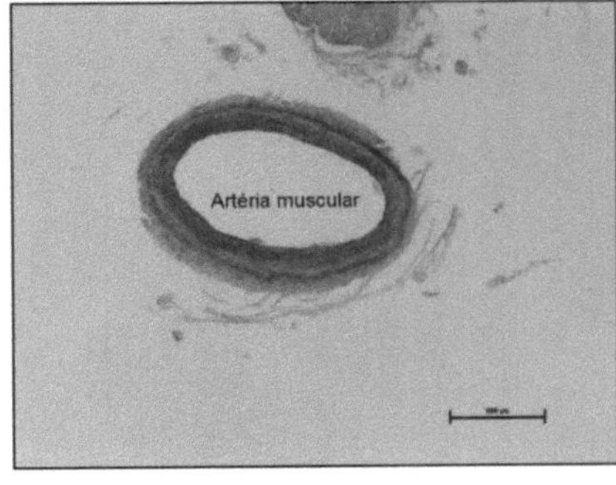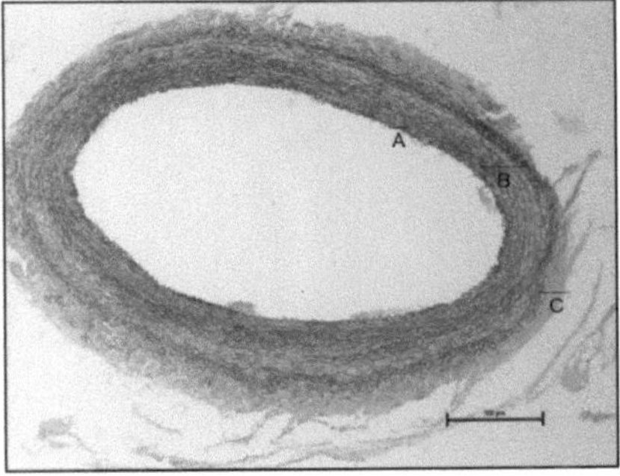

Elastic art

(A)Intimate tunic.

(B)Medium, thick tunic, composed of organized elastic fibres.

(C)Adventitious technique.

Figure 13

HISTOLOGICAL SECTIONS

VelA

HEMATOXYLIN-EOSIN STAINING TECHNIQUE

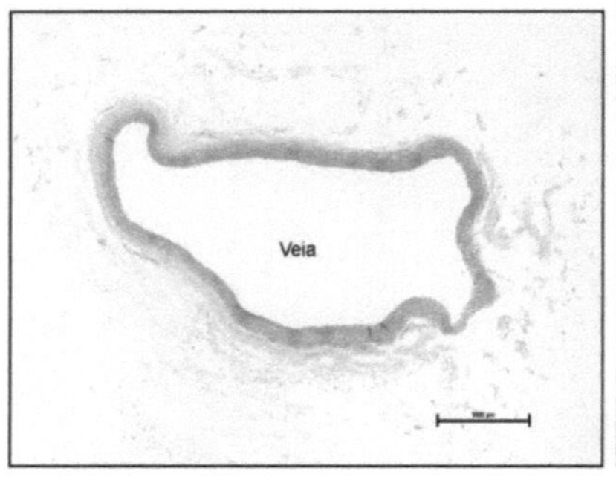
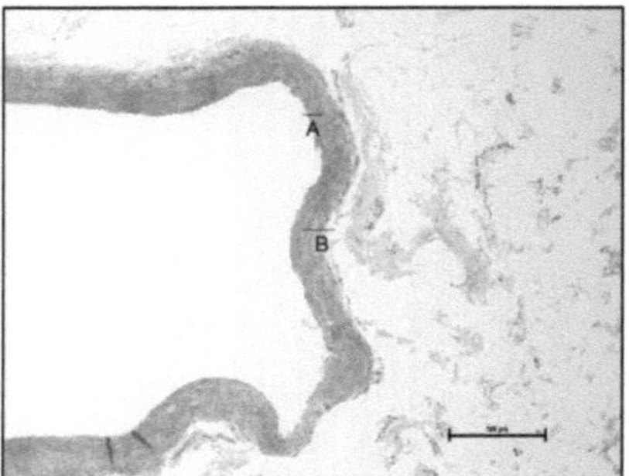

Vein

(A)Middle tonic.

(B)Adventitious tunic.

VAN GEISON STAINING TECHNIQUE

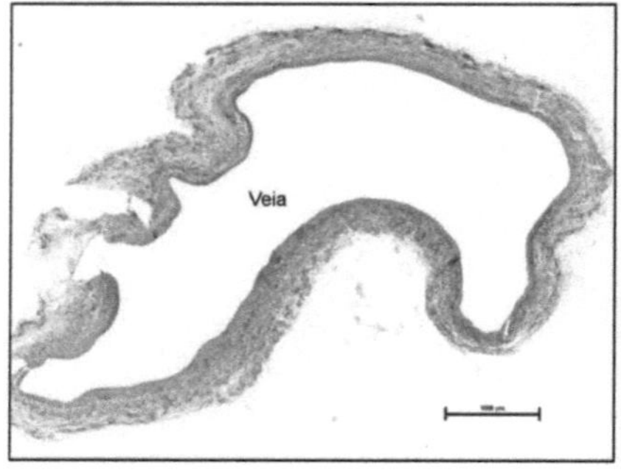
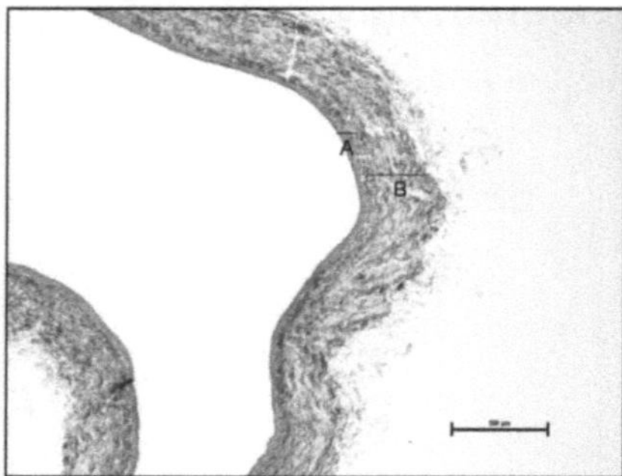

Vein

(A)Middle tonic.

(B)Adventitious tunic.

Figure 14 HISTOLOGICAL SECTIONS

CARDIAC MUSCLE AND VESSELS

HEMATOXYLIN-EOSIN STAINING TECHNIQUE

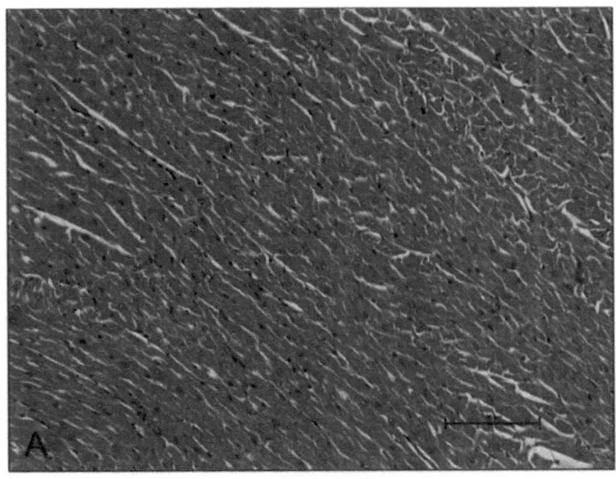

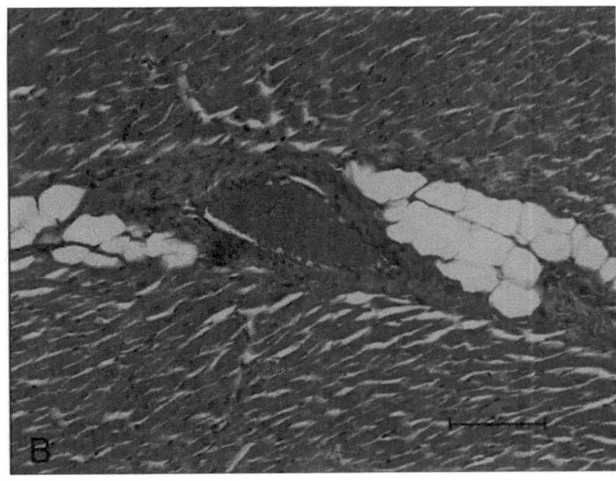

Cardiac MUSCLE

(A)Left ventricular myocardium, cross-section (20X).

(B)Congested blood vessel (20x).

1.7 Evaluation carried out with visitors using the questionnaire

A total of 264 visitors, members of the university's external and internal community, signed the attendance book for the Anatomical Exhibition of Human Hearts at the Dynamic Interdisciplinary Museum (MUDI) of the State University of Maringà (UEM). Of the 131 visitors over the age of 18, 105 (85.15%) answered the questionnaire. The sample, predominantly female (69.52%), was characterized as young adult since the average age was between 18 and 28 (40.95%) and 28 and 38 (27%). Ages between 38 and 48 and over 48 accounted for 21.9% and 9.51%, respectively.

There were no illiterate visitors or those with incomplete primary education. On the contrary, while only 6.66% were in elementary school, 25.71% were in high school, 38.09% had incomplete higher education, 10.47% had completed higher education and 19.03% had specializations, master's degrees and/or doctorates.

The visitors' knowledge of the functions of blood vessels and the heart can be seen in Figure 15.

Figure 15. Visitors' knowledge of the function of blood vessels and the heart at a scientific exhibition

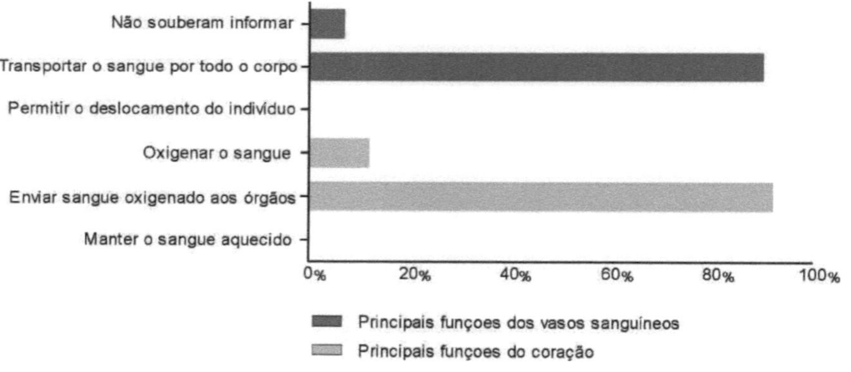

(Source: Authors, 2017).

Figure 16 shows the frequency with which the participants had consultations with cardiologists and vascular doctors as a preventative method. In addition, the visitors' family history of cardiovascular disease can be seen.

Figura 16. Knowledge of visitors to a scientific exhibition about preventive consultations and family history of diseases of the cardiovascular system

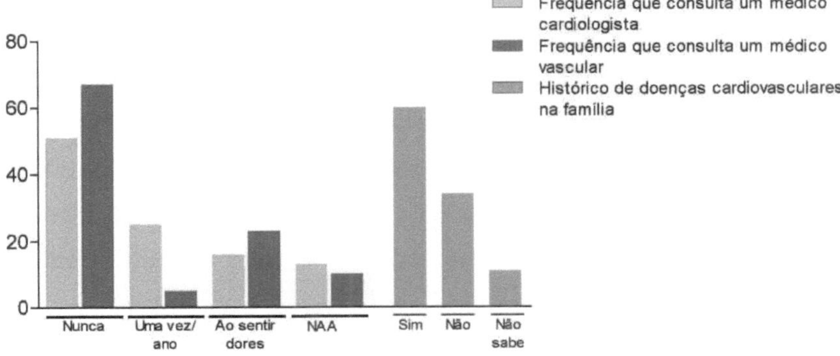

*NAA- None of the above

(Source: Authors, 2017).

Figure 17 lists the diseases that those assessed considered to be cardiovascular.

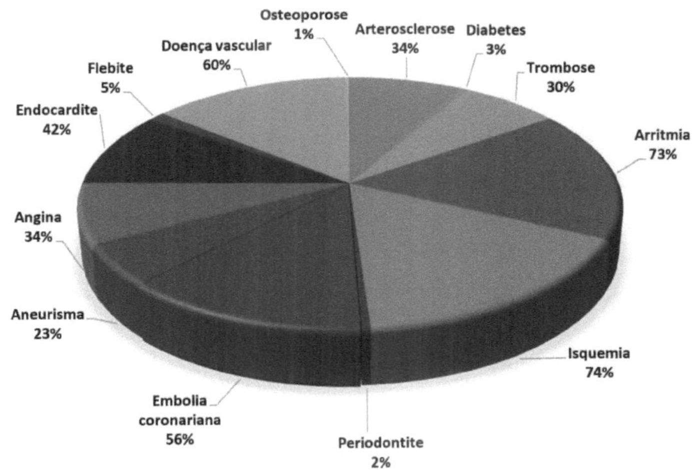

Figura 17. Diseases that visitors to a scientific exhibition considered to be cardiovascular

(Source: Authors, 2017).

When visitors were asked if they had ever received information and/or guidance on the main signs and symptoms of cardiovascular diseases, 60% of them said yes, 36% said they had never been given guidance on the subject and 4% didn't answer the question. Among those who answered positively, the main signs and symptoms (such as tiredness, chest pains and shortness of breath) were appropriately scored. In addition, participants were asked to identify the means by which they obtained this information. Personal studies were mentioned by 41.61% of those assessed, television by 30%, internet by 31.66%, medical advice by 35% and only 10% through friends and/or family. It is important to note that respondents were allowed to select more than one option.

Table 1 shows some of the signs and symptoms of heart and vascular diseases, and the percentage that those assessed identified as correlated with them.

Table 1. Participants' knowledge of the signs and symptoms of cardiovascular disease at a scientific exhibition

ALTERNATIVES	Signs and symptoms of heart disease	Signs and symptoms of vascular diseases
Chest pains, shortness of breath, headaches and palpitations	95,23%	0%
Chest pain, fever, anemia and dizziness	0,95%	0%
Fever, palpitations, body spots and convulsions	0,95%	0%
Foot pain, dizziness, coughing and shortness of breath	0,95%	0%
Yellow nails, fever, headache and dizziness	0%	0%
Pain in the legs (even at rest), reddened feet	0%	79,04%
Foot pain, cough and fever	0%	0%
High fever, flushing of the skin and headaches	0%	3,8%
Dizziness, body aches and palpitations	0%	15,23%
Reddened feet, vomiting and diarrhea	1,92%	0%
Total	100%	100%

(Source: Authors, 2017).

The participants' knowledge of the main tests that can be used to diagnose cardiovascular diseases is shown in Figure 18. An analysis of this shows that the majority of those assessed demonstrated knowledge of the tests used to diagnose cardiovascular diseases, with the electrocardiogram being the most frequently mentioned, followed by catheterization and angiography.

Figure 18. Tests used to diagnose cardiovascular diseases according to visitors to a scientific exhibition

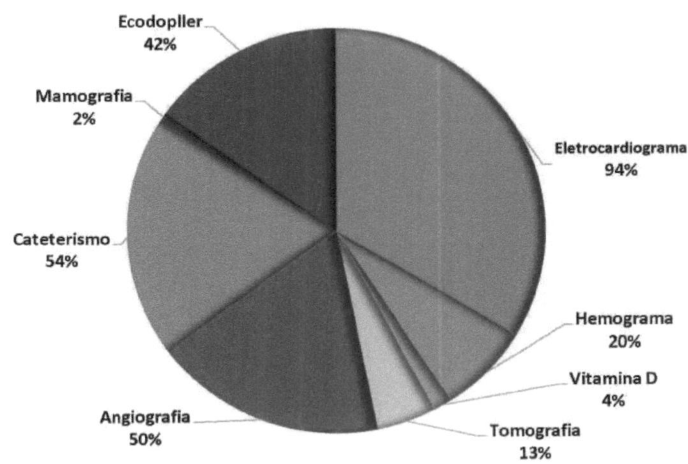

(Source: Authors, 2017).

When the participants' knowledge of the risk factors and preventive aspects of the main heart and vascular diseases was assessed, it was observed (Table 2) that the majority (84.66%) recognized obesity, smoking, a sedentary lifestyle and high blood pressure as being the most associated with the onset of these diseases. In addition, 79.04% chose the correct option for preventive measures for heart disease and 80% for vascular disease.

Table 2. Knowledge of the population assessed about risk factors and preventive measures for heart and vascular diseases.

ALTERNAOVAS	Risk factors for the onset of cardiovascular disease	The following behaviors can prevent heart disease	The following behaviors can prevent vascular diseases
Heredity, frequent sun exposure, high blood pressure and obesity.	6,66%		
Obesity, smoking, sedentary lifestyle and high blood pressure.	84,66%		
Excessive physical activity, consumption of soft drinks, smoking and diabetes.	1,98%		
Older age, female gender, smoking and frequent use of alcohol.	0,95%		

Avoid eating a lot of sugar, reading every day, drinking 2 liters of water a day and smoking.		1,90%	
Avoiding stress, running every day and having a pet		O	
Avoid stress, eat healthily, don't smoke and always monitor your cholesterol levels.		79,04%	
Monitor your cholesterol and vitamin D levels, don't smoke and eat a healthy diet.		15,03%	
Don't stay in one position for too long, eat lots of herbs and vegetables, and drink lots of hot drinks throughout the day.			7,61%
Don't consume too much sugar, salt and fat, avoid standing or sitting for too long, eat more fish and go for walks.			80%
Avoid walking or standing for a long time, consume white cams and avoid excess output, sugar and fat.			1,90%
Avoid excessive consumption of salt, sugar and fat, don't smoke and avoid physical exercise.			3,80%
Did not answer the question asked	5,73%	3,83%	10,49%
Total	100%	100%	100%

(Source: Authors, 2017).

5. Discussion

The impact of cardiovascular disease today is a constant topic of debate among health researchers. Research has therefore been carried out to reduce the incidence, morbidity and mortality of these diseases (CHAVES et al., 2015).

Specific knowledge about cardiovascular diseases makes it possible to prevent and treat them appropriately and to ensure greater longevity and quality of life for the population. In this context, one of the great challenges is to make the population scientifically and technologically literate, promoting a functional understanding of the science that is produced in universities (CARVALHO, GONZAGA and NORONHA, 2011).

Museums are suitable spaces for disseminating science since, as a means of non-formal education, they aim to disseminate and popularize knowledge in a playful and easy-to-understand way (PAULA et al., 2016). In this way, believing that the Dynamic Interdisciplinary Museum (MUDI) of the State University of Maringà (UEM) is very accessible to the general population, an anatomical exhibition of human hearts was held concomitantly with the dissemination of knowledge about cardiovascular diseases and the collection of related data.

Overall, our results showed that the interviewees had a good level of knowledge about the subject. This finding may be related to the fact that the survey was carried out in an academic environment, with a young and well-educated population. However, even with this in mind, a small proportion of those surveyed mentioned diabetes and osteoporosis as cardiovascular diseases.

The number of visits to the exhibition was considered relatively small when compared to the large number of students who attend the university and the surrounding external community. This is in line with research that indicates that a large part of the Brazilian population still does not have the habit of attending academic environments (PAULA et al., 2016). In addition, although various educational actions are developed in these non-formal educational spaces, access to knowledge is still restricted, which justifies the low attendance. A study carried out among public and private school teachers in the Baixada Fluminense region of Rio de Janeiro, for example, found that the relationship between teachers and science centers and museums is worrying, since 83% said they didn't visit these spaces and 29% said they didn't even know about them (PAULA, 2013).

Some of the results obtained in this study are worrying. This is because, although those assessed showed adequate knowledge of the functions of the heart and blood vessels, a significant proportion of them (12.38%) confused the function of the heart with that of the lungs.

In addition, although the majority (57.38%) said they had a family history of cardiovascular diseases, they did not mention preventive treatment for these diseases through routine medical consultations.

It is well known that the lack of prevention leads to greater expenditure on curative treatments. According to Vieira et al. (2016), between 2008 and 2013 in the state of Bahia alone, which has a population of 14,175,341 inhabitants, there were 82,191 hospitalizations for heart failure and 46,273 for hypertension. On the other hand, Mansur and Favarato (2016) found a drop in the mortality rate related to cardiovascular diseases in developed countries as a result of investments in prevention and easier diagnosis. Similar results were found by Vilella, Klein and Oliveira (2016) who observed a drop in the mortality rate in developed countries from the first half of the 21st century when the causes that predispose to cardiovascular diseases were previously analyzed. However, according to the authors, mortality rates were higher in men than in women and rose again after this period, suggesting that new studies and research should be carried out correlating this fact to the behavior of the population.

The participants in this study recognized obesity, a sedentary lifestyle and high blood pressure as modifiable risk factors for cardiovascular disease. In addition, they correctly identified preventive measures that could be adopted in order to avoid them, such as stress reduction, smoking cessation, sporadic monitoring of cholesterol and triglyceride levels, maintaining a healthy diet and regular physical exercise.

According to Davidson (2001), in fact, the most important risk factors for cardiovascular disease can be considered preventable, with the exception of genetic factors and chronological ageing. Thus, changes in lifestyle habits could be enough to minimize many of the damages associated with them, such as the high cost of curative treatments. However, research indicates that a large part of the Brazilian population is overweight, and obesity is responsible for the deaths of 2.8 million people a year worldwide (MARTINS, 2013). For Medeiros and colleagues (2014), another equally important risk factor is a sedentary lifestyle. According to the authors, there would be a 31% reduction in the incidence of cardiovascular diseases by implementing and improving leisure areas, sports, cycle paths and spaces for socializing at work.

The majority of the population assessed in our study recognized the main diagnostic tests for cardiovascular diseases and said that they had received guidance on the signs and symptoms of these diseases, largely through television and the internet. Similar findings were published by Muniz et al. (2012) when they reported that the *North Korelia* program in Finland managed to reduce the number of deaths in the country through educational media actions linked to sports and education personalities.

Considering the multiplicity of risk factors and the pathophysiology of cardiovascular diseases, it is believed that the adoption of healthy lifestyle habits and preventive measures can minimize the damage caused by these diseases. Thus, controlling risk factors, disseminating preventive information about these diseases and investing in medical developments that favor early diagnosis will be essential to reducing the number of hospitalizations, costs and future deaths caused by them.

6. CONCLUSION

The population evaluated had satisfactory knowledge of cardiovascular diseases in terms of their signs and symptoms, forms of diagnosis and treatment. However, those assessed were still not very aware of the preventive aspects of these diseases.

In this way, it is hoped that the profile portrayed here can contribute relevant information for the application of new public policies to be adopted preventively in order to minimize the incidence and serious consequences of cardiovascular diseases in Brazil.

7. REFERENCES

BAHIA, L.; ARAÙJO, D. V. Economic impact of obesity in Brazil. **Revista Hospital Universitàrio Pedro Ernesto**, Rio de Janeiro, v. 13, n. 1, 2014.

BESTETTI, R. B.; RESTINI, C. B.; COUTO.B. Carlos Chagas' discoveries as a backdrop for the scientific construction of chronic chagasic heart disease. **Arquivo Brasileiro de Cardiologia**, v. 107, n. 1, p. 63-70, 2016.

BESTETTI, R. B.; RESTINI, C. B.; COUTO L. B. Evolution of anatomophysiological knowledge of the cardiovascular system: from the Egyptians to Harvey. **Arquivo Brasileiro de Cardiologi,**. v. 103, n. 6, p. 538-545, 2014.

BONOW, R. O.; MANN, D. L.; ZIPES, D. P.; LIBB. P. **Tratado de Doenças Cardiovasculares**. v. 2, 6. ed. Rio de Janeiro: Editora Elsevier, 2013.

BRANDI, D. L. Acute myocardial infarction. Revista **Uniplac**, v. 5, n. 1, 2017.

BRAZIL. Ministry of Health. Strategic action plan for tackling chronic non-communicable diseases (NCDs) in Brazil 2011-2022. Brasilia: WHO, 2012.

BRASILEIRO F. G.; BOGLIOLO, L.; BITTENCOURT, A. C. L.; ALTEMANI, A. M. A. M.; BARBOSA, A. J. A.; LANA. M, A.; GUEDES, A. C. M.; HILBIG, A.; BILLIS.; TOSTA, C. E.; CARNEIRO, C, M, B. **Pathologia**. 9. ed. Rio de Janeiro: Guanabara Koogan, 2016.

BRISCHILIARI, S. C. R.; DELL AGNOLO, C. M.; GRAVENA, A. A. F.; LOPES, T. C. R.; CARVALHO, M. D. B.; PELLOSO, S. M. Chronic non-communicable diseases and association with risk factors. **Revista Brasileira de Cardiologia**, v.27, n.1 p. 531-538, 2014.

CARVALHO, M. T. S.; GONZAGA, A. M.; NORONHA, E. L. Divulgaçâo científica: dimensôes e tendências, tendências no ensino de ciências e matemàtica. **Revista Areté**, Manaus v. 4, n.7, p. 99-114, 2011.

CHAVES, C. S.; LEITAO, M. P. C.; BRAGA-JUNIOR, A. C. R.; SIRINO, A. C.

A. Identification of risk factors for cardiovascular diseases in health professionals. **Arquivos de Ciências da Saùde**, v. 22, n. 1, p. 3946, 2015.

DAVIDSON, C. **Family Health Guide**: Heart disease. special edition, 2001.

ELOI, A. F.; FELIZARDO, J. T.; SILVA NETO, J.; ROSA, M. C. B.; TARCISO, T. P.; GUIMARAES, G. C. Application of the repletion and corrosion technique to the arterial vascular system of rats (*Rattus norvegicus albinus*). SBPC Regional Meeting in Lavras, Minas Gerais, 2010.

FECHINE, B. A.; TROMPIERI, N. The aging process: The main changes that happen to the elderly over the years. **Revista Inter Science Place**, ed. 20, v.1, p. 106-194, 2012.

FERREIRA, J. S.; AYDOS, R. D. Prevalence of arterial hypertension in obese children and adolescents. **Ciência e Saùde Coletiva**, v. 15, n. 1, p. 97104, 2010.

FERRETTI, F.; GRIS, A.; MATTIELLO, D.; TEO ARRUDA, P.R.C.; SA, C. Impact of a health education program on the knowledge of elderly people about cardiovascular diseases. **Revista de Salud Pùblica**, v. 16, n. 6, p. 807-820, 2014.

HART, M.H. **The 100 Greatest Personalities in History: A Ranking of the People Who Have Most Influenced History**. 4.ed. São Paulo: Bertrand Brasil. 2001.

LEITE, I. C.; VALETE J. G.; SCHRAMM, J. M. A.; DAUMAS, R. P.; RODRIGUES, R. N.; SANTOS, M. Fâtima.; OLIVEIRA, A. F.; SILVA, R. S.; CAMPOS, M. Rodrigues.; MOTA, J. C. Burden of disease in Brazil and its regions, 2008. **Caderno Saùde Pùblica**, Rio de Janeiro, v. 31, n.7, p.15511564, jul.2015.

MACIEL, B. C.; NETO, J. A. M. **Manual de condutas clinicas cardiológicas**. v. 1. Sâo Paulo: Editora segmentos Farma, 2005.

MAIA, L. C. F. O.; CUNHA, M. B. Da pedagogicidade do cuidado ante a experiência de ser hypertenso. **Revista Interface-Comunicaçâo, Saùde, Educaçâo,** v. 18, p. 1463-1474, 2014.

MALTA, D. C.; SILVA-JÛNIOR, J. B. The strategic action plan for tackling chronic non-communicable diseases in Brazil and the definition of global targets for tackling these diseases by 2025: a review. **Epidemiologia e Serviços de Saùde,** v. 22, n.1, p. 151-164, 2013.

MANSUR, A. P. A.; FAVARATO, D. Trends in the Mortality Rate from Cardiovascular Diseases in Brazil, 1980-2012. **Arquivo Brasileiro de Cardiologia**, v. 107, n. 1, p. 20-25, 2016.

MARTINS, I. N. S. Evaluation of risk factors for cardiovascular diseases in adolescents and young adults in the federal district. 2013. Available at: http://bdm.unb.br/handle/10483/9331. Accessed on 03/Nov. 2017, 10:05.

MEDEIROS, M. S.; SACRAMENTO, D. S.; GUERREIRO, J. C. H.; ORTIZA, R. A.; FENNER, A. L. D. Cost of illness attributable to environmental factors in the city of Manaus, state of Amazonas, Brazil. **Ciência & Saùde Coletiva**, v. 19, n. 2, p. 599-608, 2014.

MUNIZ, L. C.; SHNEIDER, C. B.; SILVA, M. C. I.; MATIJASEVICH, A.; SANTOS, S. I. Cumulative behavioral risk factors for cardiovascular disease in southern Brazil. **Revista de Saùde Pùblica**, v. 46, n. 3, p. 534-542, 2012.

MUSSI, F. C.; PEREIRA, A. Pain tolerance in myocardial infarction. **Acta Paul Enferm**, v.23, n.1, p.80-87, 2010.

NETO, M. H. M. **Human Anatomy**: Dynamic Learning. 3.ed. Maringà: Clichetec, 2008.

PAULA, L. M. Museu de Ciências lugar do pùblico! A case study on the spontaneous public visiting a science museum in Rio de Janeiro. Osvaldo Cruz Foundation. Rio de Janeiro. 2013.

PAULA, L. M.; PEREIRA, G. R.; DE PAULA, L. M.; SILVA, R. C. O entorno que nãoâo vai: A case study of the non-public of a science museum in rio de janeiro. **Ensino, Saùde e Ambiente,** v. 9, n. 3, 2016.

QUINTANA, J. F.; KALIL, R. A. K. Cardiac surgery: psychological manifestations of the patient in the pre- and postoperative period. **Psicologia hospitalar,** v.10, n.2, p. 16-32, 2012.

RODRIGUES, T. M. A.; PALMEIRA, J. A. O.; MENDONÇA, J. T.; GOMES, O. M. Evolutionary study of the anatomy of coronary arteries in vertebrate species using the vinyl acetate (vinylite) modeling technique. **Revista Brasileira Cirurgia Cardiovascular,** v. 14, n. 4, p. 331-339, 1999.

SILVERTHORN, D. U. **Human Physiology**. 5.ed. Porto Alegre: ArteMed, 2010.

TRAPÉ, A. A.; SACARDO, A.; CASSIA, A.; MONTEIRO I. H.; ZAGO, A. S. Relationship between unsupervised walking and risk factors for cardiovascular disease in adults and the elderly. **Medicina,** v.47, n.2, p. 165-176, 2014.

VIEIRA, E. C.; CARDOSO, C. C. A.; MACÊDO, B. L.; DIAS, C. C. M. C. Occurrence of hospitalizations due to diseases of the circulatory system in the state of bahia. **Revista Pesquisa em Fisioterapia**, v. 6, n. 2, 2016.

VILLELA, P. Blanco.; KLEIN, C. H.; DE OLIVEIRA, G. M. M. Evolution of Mortality from Cerebrovascular and Hypertensive Diseases in Brazil between 1980 and 2012. **Hypertension**, v. 107, n. 1, p. 26-32, 2016.

8.   ANNEXES

ANNEX 1 - QUESTIONNAIRE

1.   Which of the following age groups do you currently fall into?

(   ) From 18 to 28 years old

(   ) From 28 to 38 years old

(   ) From 38 to 48 years old

(   ) From 48 to 58 years old

(   ) From 58 to 68 years old

(   ) over 68 years old

2.   What's your gender?

(   ) Male

(   ) Female

3.   What is your level of education?

(   )   Incomplete   primary education

(   )   Complete elementary school

(   )   Incomplete   high school education

(   )   Complete high school education

(   )   Higher   educationincomplete

(   )   Higher education completed

(   )   Specialization

(   )   Master

(   )   Doctorate

(   )   Post-doctorate

4.   How often do you see a cardiologist?

(   ) I've never been to a cardiologist.

(   ) I go at least once a year.

(   ) I only   go for surgical procedures.

5.   How often do you see a vascular doctor?

(   ) I've never been to a vascular doctor.

(   ) I go at least once a year.

(   ) I only go when I feel pain.

6.   Do any of   your family members   have a history of cardiovascular disease?

(   )   Yes

(   )   No

(   ) I don' t   know

7.   What is the heart's main function?

(   ) Keeping the blood warm.

(   ) Sending blood rich in oxygen and nutrients to the organs.

(   ) Oxygenate the blood.

8.   What is the main function of blood vessels?

(   ) Allowing the individual to move around in the environment.

(   ) Transporting blood throughout the body.

(   ) To oxygenate the blood.

9.   Which diseases below do you consider to be cardiovascular diseases?

(   )   Atherosclerosis

(   )   Diabetes

(   )   Thrombosis

( )   Pneumonia

(   )Myocardial ischemia

( )   Arrhythmia

( )   Periodontitis

( )   Coronary embolism

( )   Aneurysm

( )   Angina

( )   Endocarditis

( )   Phlebitis

( )   Psoriasis

( )   Peripheral vascular disease

( )   Osteoporosis

10. Have you ever received any advice on the main signs?

and symptoms of cardiovascular disease?

(   ) Yes

(   ) No

11. If the answer to the above question was **YES**, please give a brief

describe the main signs and symptoms of cardiovascular diseases and then answer question 12. If your answer above is **NO**, go to question 13.

12. How did you obtain the information described above?

( )   On television

( )   On the internet

( )   With friends or family

( )   For my personal   studies

(   ) On medical advice

(   ) Another source. Which source? _________________________________

13. Which of the following are signs and symptoms of heart disease?

(   ) Chest pains, shortness of breath, headaches and palpitations.

(   ) Chest pain, fever, anemia and dizziness.

(   ) Fever, palpitations, spots on the body and convulsions.

(   ) Leg pain, dizziness, coughing and shortness of breath.

(   ) Yellow nails, fever, headache and dizziness.

14. Which of the following are signs and symptoms of vascular diseases?

(   ) Pain in the legs (even at rest), cold and red feet.

(   ) Pain in the legs, cough and fever.

(   ) High fever, flushing of the legs and headaches.

(   ) Dizziness, body aches and palpitations.

(   ) Cold, red feet, vomiting and diarrhea.

15. What is a heart attack or myocardial infarction?

(   ) Altered conduction of electrical impulses by the heart.

(   ) Abnormal smallness of the heart, associated with mental deficiency.

(   ) Process of necrosis of part of the heart muscle due to lack of adequate
supply of nutrients and oxygen.

(   ) Inflammation of the heart caused by infectious agents.

16. What is atherosclerosis?

(   ) A disease that primarily affects the heart muscle.

(   ) Heart disease present from birth.

(   ) Disease related to a drop in calcium absorption.

(   ) A disease related to the deposition of fat on the wall of blood vessels.

17. Which of the following are the main risk factors for cardiovascular disease?

(   ) Heredity, frequent sun exposure, high blood pressure and obesity.

(   ) Obesity, smoking, sedentary lifestyle and high blood pressure.

(   ) Excessive physical   activity, consumption of soft drinks, smoking and diabetes.

(   ) Older   age, female gender, smoking and frequent use of alcohol.

18. Which of the tests listed below can be used to diagnose cardiovascular diseases? (You can check as many boxes as you like):

(   )   Electrocardiogram

(   )   Blood count

(   )   Vitamin   D dosage

(   )   Tomography

(   )   Angiography

(   )   Catheterization

(   )   Mammography

(   )   Ecodopller

19. Which of the following behaviors can prevent heart disease? (   )

 Avoid eating too much sugar, read every day, drink 2 liters of water

a day and smoking.

(   ) Avoid stress, run every day and have a pet.

(   ) Avoid stress, eat healthily, don't smoke and always monitor your cholesterol levels.

(   ) Monitor your cholesterol and vitamin D levels, don't smoke and eat a healthy diet.

20. Which of the following behaviors can prevent vascular disease.

(   ) Don't stay in one position for too long, eat lots of fruit and vegetables, and drink plenty of hot drinks throughout the day.

(   ) Don't consume too much sugar, salt and fat, avoid standing or sitting for too long, eat more fish and walk.

(   ) Avoid walking or standing for too long, eat white meat and avoid excess salt, sugar and fat.

(   ) Avoid excessive consumption of salt, sugar and fat, don't smoke and avoid physical exercise.

ANNEX 2

TERM OF FREE AND INFORMED CONSENT (TCLE)

We would like to invite you to participate in the research entitled **"Analysis of the knowledge of a population visiting a scientific exhibition about cardiovascular diseases"** as part of the specialization course in Human Anatomy and Histology, and is supervised by Professor Dr. Carmen Patricia Barbosa of the State University of Maringà (UEM).

The aim of this survey is to assess the level of knowledge of some visitors to a Human Anatomy exhibition about the main cardiovascular diseases. For this, your participation is very important and must be completely voluntary. The ICF will be presented and explained to you and after confirming your voluntary consent, you will be instructed to answer an investigative questionnaire with the aim of analyzing your knowledge of factors related to the main cardiovascular diseases (such as causes, main signs and symptoms, diagnostic methods and preventive factors). Please note that only randomly selected visitors over the age of 18, of both sexes, will take part in the survey.

The questionnaires should be completed at the time of the visit and handed in to the researchers as soon as they are finished. After the questionnaires have been completed, the participants in the research and all visitors to the exhibition will be given the opportunity to see theoretical and practical demonstrations of the circulatory system and the main aspects of cardiovascular disease. For this purpose, specially prepared anatomical pieces and *banners* with appropriate information and illustrations will be used.

Please be aware that risks may occur when filling in the questionnaire, such as personal discomfort due to viewing the pieces or even due to the weather or personal health aspects. However, in any of these situations, immediate assistance will be provided and, if necessary, referral will be made to specialized help. In addition, we would like to make it clear that your participation is completely voluntary and that you can refuse to take part or even withdraw at any time without this entailing any burden or harm to you. As no expenses are foreseen for carrying out this study, there will be no financial compensation. We also inform you that the information will only be used for the purposes of this research and will be treated with the utmost secrecy and confidentiality, in order to preserve your identity. The results may therefore be published in scientific journals in the field in the future and, if you are interested, you can find out the final results of the study at any time by contacting one of the researchers.

The expected benefit of this study is to provide the population with information on the most relevant aspects of the main cardiovascular diseases, such as definition, main signs and symptoms, forms of diagnosis, available treatments, as well as clarification on risk factors and prevention.

If you have any further questions or require further clarification, you can contact us at the addresses below or contact the UEM Research Ethics Committee (COPEP), whose address is given in this document. This form must be completed in two copies of equal content, one of which, duly completed and signed, will be given to you. In addition to the signatures in the specific fields by the researcher and by you, we ask that you initial all the pages of this document. This must be done by both of us (the researcher and you as the subject) in such a way as to guarantee access to the entire document.

Me,

...(full name of the research subject) declare that I have been duly informed and agree to **voluntarily** participate in the research coordinated by Professor Dr. Carmen Patricia Barbosa.

Date: _______________________________

Signature or fingerprint

I, Sandra Regina Magalhâes, declare that I have provided all the information regarding the above research project.

Date: _______________________________

Researcher's signature

CONTACT ADDRESSES

Carmen Patricia Barbosa

Avenida Colombo, n° 5.790, Jardim Universitàrio, CEP 87020-900, Maringà-

PR; Phone (44) 3011-6008

E-mail: carmemmecl @gmail.com

COPEP/UEM - Permanent Committee for Ethics in Research Involving Human Beings

UEM Human Resources

Maringà State University.

Colombo Avenue, 5790. UEM Headquarters Campus.

UEM Central Library (BCE) block.

ZIP CODE 87020-900. Maringà-Pr. Tel: (44) 3261-4444

E-mail:copep@uem.br

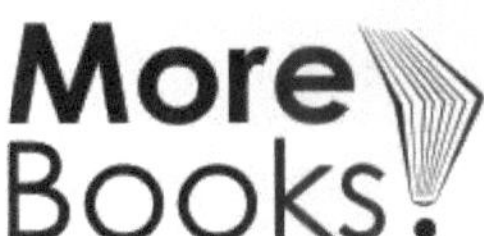

More Books!

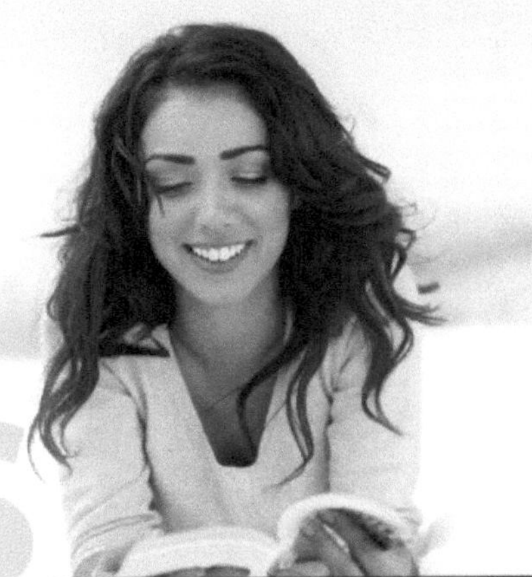

yes

I want morebooks!

Buy your books fast and straightforward online - at one of world's fastest growing online book stores! Environmentally sound due to Print-on-Demand technologies.

Buy your books online at

www.morebooks.shop

Kaufen Sie Ihre Bücher schnell und unkompliziert online – auf einer der am schnellsten wachsenden Buchhandelsplattformen weltweit! Dank Print-On-Demand umwelt- und ressourcenschonend produzi ert.

Bücher schneller online kaufen

www.morebooks.shop

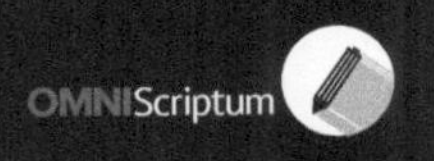

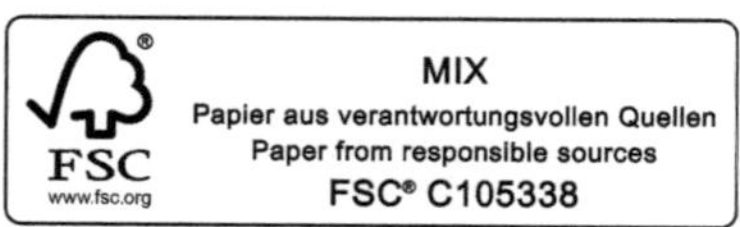

Printed by Books on Demand GmbH, Norderstedt / Germany